THE DIFFERENT BETWEEN STRENGHT TRAINING AND EXERCISE

THE EYE OPENER

CYRIL LAKES

Contents

CHAPTER ONE

INTRODUCTION

Exercise and strength training are essential parts of a comprehensive fitness program, each providing special advantages for overall physical health and performance. Despite the fact that the terms are frequently used synonymously, they refer to different types of physical activity with different goals and purposes. We'll go over the main distinctions between exercise and strength training in this introduction, as well as how each promotes endurance, strength, and general fitness.

An explanation of the benefits of physical activity for general fitness and health

Engaging in physical activity is essential for enhancing general health and fitness in a variety of domains related to wellbeing. This explains why it's important:

Cardiovascular Health: Cardiovascular health is enhanced by regular physical activity, such as aerobic exercise, which fortifies the heart. It lessens the risk of heart disease, stroke, and other cardiovascular disorders by lowering blood pressure, lowering LDL cholesterol, and raising HDL cholesterol.

Weight management: When paired with a balanced diet, physical activity helps people burn calories and maintain a healthy body weight or reach their weight loss objectives. By improving metabolism, maintaining lean muscle mass, and encouraging fat loss, it lowers the risk of obesity and related conditions like metabolic syndrome and type 2 diabetes.

Musculoskeletal Health: Weight-bearing activities and strength training contribute to the development and maintenance of strong bones, muscles, and joints. Frequent exercise lowers the risk of osteoporosis, sarcopenia, and osteoarthritis by improving joint flexibility and stability, building muscle strength and endurance, and increasing bone density.

Mental Health and Well-Being: Engaging in physical activity provides several advantages for mental health, such as lowering feelings of stress, anxiety, and depression. Exercise improves mood, sleep quality, and cognitive performance by triggering the production of endorphins, which are neurotransmitters that encourage emotions of contentment and relaxation.

Enhanced Energy: Physical activity on a regular basis boosts energy levels and lessens exhaustion and sluggishness. greater vigor, productivity, and general quality of life are the results of its improved circulation, improved oxygen delivery to tissues, greater brain activity, and increased metabolism.

Disease Prevention: Engaging in physical activity is linked to a decreased chance of developing chronic illnesses and ailments, such as osteoporosis, type 2 diabetes, depression, anxiety disorders, and specific cancers (such as breast and colon cancer). It supports immune system performance and general disease resistance in addition to regulating insulin sensitivity, inflammation, and blood sugar levels.

Quality of Life and Longevity: Studies continually demonstrate that people who regularly participate in physical exercise have longer lifespans and better quality of life than inactive people. Engaging in physical activity as one ages improves functional ability, mobility, and independence while lowering the risk of dying young from all causes.

Social engagement and Community: Whether through team sports, group fitness sessions, or outdoor leisure activities, engaging in physical activity frequently entails social engagement and community building. Developing connections and exchanging stories with people who share similar interests can promote a feeling of support, camaraderie, and belonging, all of which are critical for one's mental and emotional well.

Engaging in physical activity is crucial for maintaining total health and fitness, which includes mental, social, and physical aspects of well-being. People can experience a healthier, happier, and more fulfilled life and reap the many advantages of physical activity by embracing a variety of activities that suit individual tastes and skills and including regular exercise into daily routines.

Strength training definition

By gradually overloading the muscles with resistance, strength training also referred to as resistance training or weight training—is a type of exercise intended to increase muscular strength, power, and endurance. It entails using resistance-training exercises with bodyweight, free weights, weight machines, or resistance bands to push the muscles and encourage adaptations that result in bigger, stronger, more functionally capable muscles.

By repeatedly contracting muscles against resistance, strength training aims to cause hypertrophy, or the growth and expansion of muscle fibers. During activity, muscle fibers sustain microtears that are subsequently repaired and rebuilt into larger, stronger structures during rest and recovery periods. Regular strength training improves overall body composition, metabolic rate, and functional performance over time in addition to increasing muscle strength, endurance, and power.

Exercises that focus on certain muscle groups or movement patterns, such squats, deadlifts, bench presses, rows, and overhead presses, are examples of strength training exercises. These workouts are adaptable and customizable based on personal preferences, objectives, and fitness levels since they can be done with a variety of tools and modalities. Different training variables, such as volume, frequency, intensity, and exercise selection, can be included in strength training regimens to maximize muscle growth, strength increases, and performance enhancements.

Beyond just developing muscles, strength training has many other advantages such as increased bone density, joint stability, and functional mobility; it also improves body composition, metabolic health, and general physical performance. It is a useful part of a comprehensive exercise program that may be done by people of different ages, skill levels, and fitness levels, from novices to professional athletes. Strength training can be a safe, entertaining, and effective strategy to improve physical health, functional ability, and quality of life with the right technique, progression, and supervision.

What Exercise Means

Any organized physical activity done to maintain or enhance physical fitness, general health, or overall well-being is referred to as exercise. It entails deliberate, planned body motions that activate different muscle groups and energy systems, resulting in physiological changes and positive health effects.

Important aspects of exercise consist of:

Structured Activity: Exercise entails deliberate, planned motions or activities carried out with the aim of enhancing physical fitness or reaching particular health objectives. It frequently adheres to a set schedule or program made to focus on particular aspects of fitness, like muscular strength, flexibility, balance, or cardiovascular endurance.

Physical Effort: Engaging in exercise calls for more physical effort and exertion than one might do in regular life. It puts more strain on the body's systems, forcing the respiratory, musculoskeletal, and cardiovascular systems to advance and adapt to meet rising demands.

Exercise usually consists of repeated motions or activities carried out regularly over an extended period of time in order to meet specific fitness or health objectives. To fully reap the benefits of exercise, one must be consistent in their efforts. Regular exercisers experience progressive gains in their physical and general well-being.

Diverse Modalities: Exercise can be performed in a variety of ways, such as bodyweight exercises, functional fitness training, strength training (weightlifting, resistance training), flexibility exercises (yoga, stretching), and aerobic activities (walking, running, cycling). Exercise modalities might differ depending on personal preferences, objectives, and physical capabilities.

Benefits of Exercise for Your Health and Fitness: Exercise improves your cardiovascular health, your muscles' strength and endurance, your flexibility and mobility, your metabolic health, your mood, your stress level, and your cognitive function, among many other physical, mental, and emotional advantages.

All things considered, physical activity is an essential part of a healthy lifestyle and is critical for enhancing overall quality of life, preventing chronic diseases, and fostering physical fitness. People can gain the various benefits of physical activity and reach their fitness and health objectives by picking meaningful and enjoyable activities to include into their routines, in addition to regular exercise.

CHAPTER TWO

Strength Training Advantages

Numerous advantages of strength training exist for general well-being, functional ability, and physical health. Key advantages of strength training include the following:

Strength training promotes muscle hypertrophy and growth, which results in an increase in both muscle mass and strength. This boosts mobility, stability, and functional capacity in addition to improving physical appearance throughout daily activities.

Increased muscle Strength and Power: Consistent strength training increases muscle strength and power, enabling people to carry out tasks more easily and effectively. Gaining strength can help you perform better in sports, leisure pursuits, and everyday tasks like carrying groceries, climbing stairs, and lifting objects.

Enhanced Metabolic Rate: Because sustaining lean muscle mass requires more energy, strength training raises metabolic rate even while you're at rest. This can encourage calorie burning and fat oxidation, which can aid in weight reduction, weight management, and improvements in body composition.

Bone Health: Strength training activities, especially those involving weightlifting and resistance training, increase bone mineralization and density, which lowers the incidence of fractures and osteoporosis. Strength training increases bone growth and remodeling by putting stress on the bones, which over time results in stronger, denser bones.

Joint Health and Stability: Strength training improves joint stability and lowers the chance of injury by strengthening the muscles, tendons, and ligaments surrounding joints. By enhancing joint mobility and function, it can help reduce joint pain and stiffness brought on by diseases like rheumatoid arthritis and osteoarthritis.

Better Posture and Balance: Exercises focusing on strength training target all of the body's muscles, including those involved in maintaining balance and posture. Strength training helps with posture, spinal alignment, and balance. It also lowers the chance of falls and accidents by strengthening the muscles in the core, back, and stabilizing areas.

Enhanced Functional Capacity: Strength training increases muscle endurance, coordination, and movement efficiency, which boosts functional capacity and performance in daily life tasks. Greater mobility, independence, and self-assurance in carrying out activities like lifting, bending, reaching, and walking can result from this.

Chronic Illness Management: Research has demonstrated the advantages of strength training in the treatment of a number of chronic illnesses, including as osteoporosis, diabetes, arthritis, and cardiovascular disease. Along with lowering symptoms like pain and exhaustion, it enhances insulin sensitivity, blood sugar regulation, cardiovascular health, and joint function.

Advantages for Mental Health: Strength training improves mental health and wellbeing by lowering stress, anxiety, and depressive symptoms. Exercise improves cognitive performance, emotional control, and self-esteem by releasing endorphins, neurotransmitters that encourage emotions of enjoyment and relaxation.

Quality of Life and lifespan: Research indicates that maintaining muscle strength and function as we age is crucial for preserving independence, vitality, and general healthspan. Strength training has been linked to both increased lifespan and quality of life.

All things considered, strength training is an important part of a comprehensive fitness program that has several advantages for general health, functional ability, and well-being. People can benefit from strength training's many benefits and improve their quality of life and health by adding regular strength training into their routines and gradually pushing their muscles with resistance exercises.

Advantages of Physical Activity

There are numerous advantages to exercise for mental, emotional, and physical health. Here are a few main advantages of consistent exercise:

Better Cardiovascular Health: Exercise lowers blood pressure and lowers the risk of heart disease, stroke, and other cardiovascular disorders by strengthening the heart and enhancing circulation.

Weight management: When paired with a balanced diet, regular physical exercise helps control body weight by burning calories and encouraging fat loss, which can assist achieve weight loss or maintenance goals.

Enhanced Muscular Strength and Endurance: Exercise, especially resistance training and strength training, improves functional capacity and performance in sports and daily activities by building muscle strength, endurance, and power.

Improved Bone Health: Resistance and weight-bearing activities increase bone strength and density, which lowers the risk of osteoporosis and fractures, particularly in older persons.

Increased Range of Motion and Flexibility: Stretching and flexibility exercises increase range of motion, flexibility, and joint mobility. This lowers the risk of injury and improves general physical function.

Improved Metabolic Health: Regular exercise lowers the risk of type 2 diabetes and metabolic syndrome by boosting lipid metabolism, raising insulin sensitivity, and controlling blood sugar levels.

Stress Reduction: Exercise is a natural way to reduce stress by lowering cortisol and other stress hormone levels and encouraging the release of endorphins, which are neurotransmitters that improve mood and encourage relaxation.

Mood Enhancement: Exercise improves mental health by lessening the signs and symptoms of anxiety, depression, and mood disorders. It also boosts confidence, self-worth, and general emotional well-being.

Better Cognitive Function: Exercise increases brain activity and improves memory, focus, and cognitive function. It also lowers the risk of age-related cognitive illnesses like dementia and Alzheimer's disease as well as cognitive decline.

Improved Sleep Quality: People who exercise regularly sleep longer and with better quality, which enables them to go to sleep earlier, wake up feeling more rested and energised.

Increased Vitality and Productivity: Exercise increases vitality and productivity throughout the day by enhancing circulation, oxygen delivery, and metabolic rate. It also lowers sensations of exhaustion and lethargy.

Social Connection: Taking part in team sports, outdoor activities, or group exercise classes encourages social interaction, community involvement, and social support, which in turn promotes a sense of camaraderie, belonging, and connection with others.

Exercise is crucial for preserving and enhancing one's physical and mental health as well as one's general quality of life. People can enjoy the many health and fitness benefits of exercise and reach their goals by making regular physical activity a part of their routines and selecting activities they find meaningful.

Techniques for Strength Training

Strength training is a broad term for a variety of exercises and strategies meant to increase muscle growth, strength, and endurance. The following are a few popular strength training techniques:

Free Weights: Medicine balls, dumbbells, barbells, and kettlebells are examples of free weights that are useful equipment for strength training. They make it possible to perform a variety of exercises that focus on various muscle groups and movement patterns. Exercises with free weights strengthen functional strength and activate stabilizing muscles.

Machine-Based Training: By using preset movement patterns, strength training machines offer directed resistance. These machines, which are frequently seen in gyms and training facilities, provide a secure setting where newcomers may learn correct lifting techniques and target particular muscle regions.

workouts with Your Own Weight: Bodyweight workouts help you develop your strength and muscle endurance by using your own body weight as resistance. Exercises like planks, burpees, lunges, squats, and push-ups are a few examples. People of all fitness levels can conduct bodyweight workouts anywhere with the least amount of equipment needed.

Resistance Bands: To increase the resistance in strength training activities, resistance bands are elastic bands with different thicknesses and resistance levels. They help with mobility and flexibility exercises and can be used to target certain muscles by providing constant tension throughout the range of motion.

Functional Training: To increase total functional capacity and performance, functional training emphasizes movements that resemble real-life activities. It uses multi-joint, multi-planar movements that work several muscle groups at once, improving proprioception, balance, and coordination.

Plyometrics: Plyometric exercises are quick, explosive motions that make use of the muscle's stretch-shortening cycle to enhance strength, speed, and agility. Box jumps, depth jumps, jump squats, and medicine ball throws are a few examples. Athletes frequently employ plyometrics to improve their performance in sports.

Isometric Training: This type of exercise entails maintaining a static posture or tensing your muscles without moving them against a resistance or immovable object. Exercises that are isometric are useful for increasing muscle endurance and strength at particular joint angles.

High-intensity interval training, or HIIT, alternates short bursts of high-intensity exercise with low-intensity recovery or rest intervals. Intense work intervals and recovery intervals are alternated to optimize metabolic rate, cardiovascular conditioning, and calorie burn while adding strength training activities.

Strength training exercises are performed back-to-back in a circuit training session with little to no rest in between sets. It works a variety of muscle groups and quickly produces benefits for strength and cardiovascular health.

Periodization: To maximize muscle growth, strength gains, and performance while avoiding plateaus and overtraining, periodization entails gradually changing training variables like volume, frequency, and intensity over time. To accomplish particular training objectives, it usually entails segmenting training into phases, such as hypertrophy, strength, and power phases.

Through the integration of various strength training techniques into a comprehensive fitness regimen, individuals can enhance their muscle strength, endurance, hypertrophy, and functional ability to help them achieve their fitness and health objectives. To reduce the chance of injury and optimize results, it's critical to select training techniques that complement personal preferences, objectives, and physical capabilities while guaranteeing appropriate technique, progression, and recuperation.

Exercise Techniques

A wide range of activities aiming at enhancing physical fitness, health, and well-being are included in the category of exercise. Here are a few typical workout techniques:

Exercise that raises the heart and breathing rates steadily is referred to as aerobic exercise, sometimes called as cardiovascular or cardio exercise. Walking, running, cycling, swimming, dancing, and aerobic classes are a few examples. Cardiovascular health, endurance, and general fitness are all enhanced by aerobic exercise.

Strength Training: To challenge and strengthen muscles, bones, and connective tissues, strength training uses resistance. It can be done with body weight exercises (squats, push-ups), resistance bands, weight machines, and free weights (barbells, dumbbells). Muscular strength, endurance, and functional ability are all enhanced by strength training.

Exercises for increasing joint range of motion, muscle elasticity, and general flexibility are referred to as flexibility training. Tai chi, yoga, Pilates, and stretching exercises are a few examples. Improved posture, balance, and less muscle stress are all benefits of flexibility exercise.

Training for Balance: Balance workouts focus on the body's capacity to sustain equilibrium and stability. They entail exercises that test proprioception and balance, like heel-to-toe walking, standing on one leg, and utilizing stability balls and balancing boards.

CHAPTER THREE

Enhancing coordination, improving functional movement patterns, and preventing falls are all benefits of balance training.

Functional Training: To increase overall functional capacity, functional training places an emphasis on movements that replicate real-life activities. It consists of multijoint, multiplanar movements that work several muscle groups at once. Strength, mobility, stability, and coordination are improved by functional training, which benefits both daily tasks and athletic performance.

High-intensity interval training, or HIIT, alternates short bursts of high-intensity exercise with low-intensity recovery or rest intervals. Intense work intervals and recuperation intervals are alternated to optimize metabolic rate, cardiovascular conditioning, and calorie burn. Aerobic workouts, strength training exercises, or a mix of the two can be a part of HIIT.

Group Exercise programs: Taught by licensed instructors, group exercise programs provide planned exercises in a group environment. Specific exercise modalities like aerobics, cycling, weight training, dance, or mind-body exercises like Pilates and yoga may be the emphasis of the classes. Exercise variation, social support, and incentive are all provided by group fitness classes.

Outdoor Activities: You can get physical exercise while taking in the scenery and the great outdoors by participating in outdoor activities like hiking, jogging, cycling, swimming, kayaking, or sports. Engaging in outdoor activities offers advantages for mental and cardiovascular health as well as stress alleviation.

Recreational Sports: Playing sports and activities for fun, including tennis, volleyball, basketball, soccer, golf, or soccer, is a great way to keep active and become in shape. Recreational sports provide skill development, strength training, and aerobic exercise in a relaxed or competitive environment.

Exercises for the Mind-Body: These exercises concentrate on combining the mental and physical facets of health and wellbeing. In order to encourage relaxation, stress reduction, and mind-body awareness, some examples of these activities are yoga, Pilates, tai chi, and qigong. These practices incorporate physical postures, breathing exercises, and mindfulness exercises.

People can enjoy the many advantages of regular physical activity and enhance their overall physical fitness, health, and well-being by combining a range of exercise techniques into a balanced fitness regimen. Selecting activities that suit personal interests, preferences, and objectives is crucial, taking into account physical capabilities, fitness level, and resource availability. Furthermore, integrating several exercise modalities can offer a comprehensive approach to fitness that takes into account numerous facets of functional ability and physical health.

A Comparative Analysis of Strength Training and Exercise

There are a few things to bear in mind when comparing strength training to general exercise because each has different uses and advantages. Here are some crucial things to remember:

Specificity of Goals: While exercise includes a wider range of activities aimed at increasing general fitness, health, and well-being, strength training is primarily focused on improving muscle strength, power, and hypertrophy. If someone is choosing between strength training and general exercise, they should think about their individual goals and objectives.

muscular Adaptations: Progressive overloading, which is a component of strength training, promotes muscular hypertrophy and gradually grows larger and stronger muscles. While general exercise improves cardiovascular health, endurance, flexibility, and functional capacity, it may not stimulate muscle growth and strength development to the same extent.

Tools and Equipment: Bodyweight exercises, resistance bands, weight machines, and free weights are examples of the types of specialized equipment that are frequently used for strength training. For those who do not have access to a gym or specialized training equipment, general exercise is more accessible and convenient because it can incorporate a variety of activities with little to no equipment.

Intensity and Load: To challenge muscles and promote changes in strength and hypertrophy, strength training usually entails lifting larger weights or resistance. A combination of low- to moderate-intensity exercises, such swimming, cycling, or walking, can be used as general exercise. These exercises prioritize cardiovascular health and endurance above the development of maximum strength.

Training Volume and Frequency: Structured resistance exercises that focus on particular muscle groups are frequently necessary for strength training, along with sufficient rest and recuperation in between sessions. When it comes to frequency and volume, general exercise can be more adaptable, enabling people to participate in various activities according to their fitness level, schedule, and preferences.

Progression and Periodization: To maximize muscle growth and strength gains, strength training regimens frequently incorporate methodical progression and periodization, which involves gradually modifying training variables including volume, frequency, and intensity. Even while general exercise may not use the same planned progression approach, regular involvement can nevertheless improve general health and fitness.

Personal Preferences and Enjoyment: In the end, personal preferences, interests, and enjoyment may determine whether to choose strength training or more broad exercise. While some people might like the diversity and flexibility of general exercise activities like hiking, yoga, or group fitness classes, others might prefer the regulated discipline of strength training and the challenge of lifting heavy weights.

Complementary Methods: Many people find that adding both strength training and regular exercise to their fitness regimens is beneficial. These two types of exercise are not mutually exclusive. Strength training can offer a well-rounded approach to fitness that addresses several aspects of health and well-being when combined with cardiovascular exercise, flexibility training, and other physical activities.

Strength training and regular exercise provide significant advantages for overall health, physical fitness, and well-being. People should think about their own objectives, tastes, and situations when choosing which strategy to use first or how to combine the two into a well-rounded exercise regimen. Getting advice from a healthcare specialist or fitness expert can help people create customized workout regimens that meet their needs and objectives.

Summary

In summary, although both strength training and general exercise enhance general health and fitness, they have different functions and advantages. While general exercise includes a wider range of activities targeted at increasing cardiovascular health, endurance, flexibility, and functional ability, strength training concentrates on improving muscular strength, power, and hypertrophy through progressive resistance training.

In order to promote muscular growth and strength development, strength training entails specialized techniques and approaches that are frequently performed using resistance training equipment such free weights, machines, or bodyweight exercises. In order to accomplish particular strength and hypertrophy goals, it places a strong emphasis on targeted muscle responses, systematic progression, and progressive overload.

Conversely, general exercise includes a wide range of exercises and methods, such as functional motions, cardiovascular exercise, flexibility training, and balance exercises. Without necessarily emphasizing on maximal strength growth, it improves total fitness, health, and well-being through exercises that enhance cardiovascular health, mobility, flexibility, and functional capacity.

The decision between strength training and general exercise ultimately comes down to personal tastes, circumstances, and ambitions. While general exercise activities like walking, cycling, or group fitness courses are more accessible and versatile, some people may prioritize strength training due to its benefits for muscular strength, size, and power.

Whichever method is selected, adding strength training and general exercise to a comprehensive fitness regimen can have a positive impact on overall health, physical fitness, and quality of life. A balanced approach to fitness and well-being can be ensured by working with a healthcare provider or fitness professional to create customized exercise plans that meet individual tastes and goals.

THE END